The Manual For The Medical Management Of Chronic Sinusitis

A Holistic Approach

Andrew Pugliese, MD

First published in The United States in 2024 by The Nation publishers

17777 Center Court Drive Suite 600, 111 West Ocean Blvd. Long Beach, CA 90802, Unites States

https://www.thenationpublishers.com/

Our books may be purchased in bulk for promotional, educational, or business use.

Please contact The Nation Publishers at +1 562 579-4476, or by email at support@thenationpublishers.com

First Edition December 2024

To Pietro and Natalina Pugliese. You braved a new world, a new language, and a new way of life so we could have a better one.

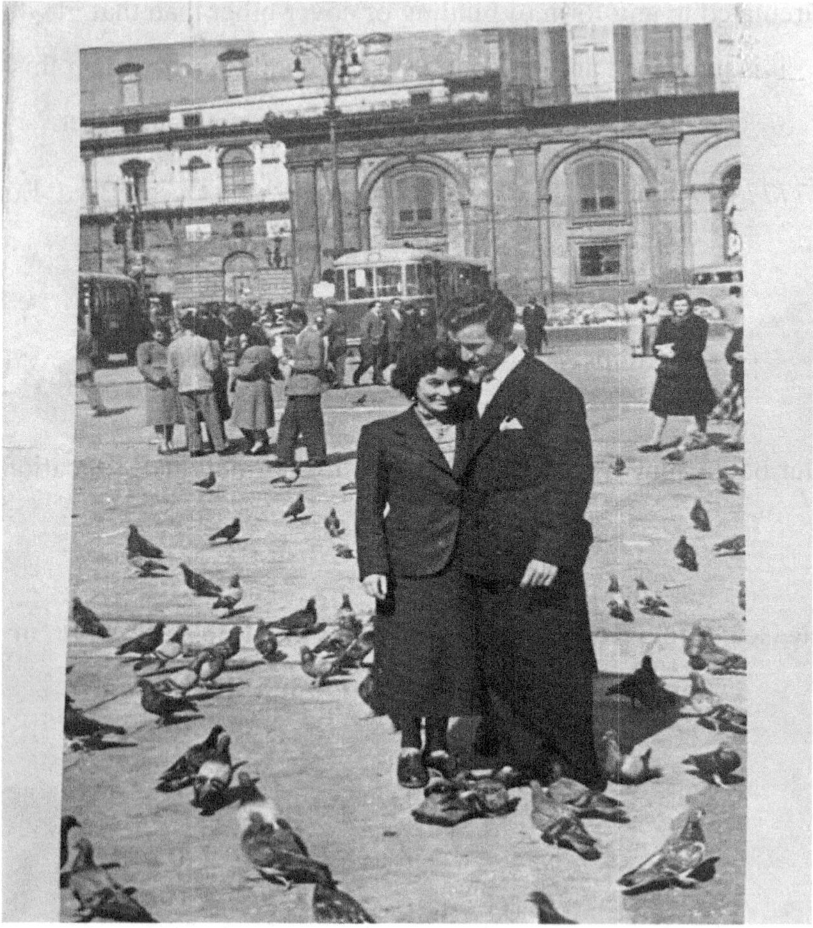

Acknowledgment

There are many people that need to be acknowledged for bringing about this book. There are too many to address individually, but first, I would like to start with the families. The Pugliese family is a large and eclectic group who don't always see eye to eye, but will always be there for you. From the oldest, who is eighty-eight, to the youngest, who is two months, but especially my wife and best friend Sandra, and our wonderful children - all five of them, Ellen, Alex, Abby, Kassandra, and Andrew, plus our two grandchildren, Jack and Gio. Your support for me as a physician, brother, uncle, nephew, cousin, and friend was always there and continues today. Thank you.

Next is the IDC family. For almost thirty years you have always been supportive of me, even those that have moved on either to retirement like Marva and Bill or to other positions; Cheryl, Tabitha to name a few. In all this time, we have taken on many challenging patients that many other clinicians had given up on. Over the years, the compliments I have received about you all make the hard days worthwhile. Thank you for all your support, for always having my best interests at heart, and for the care and professionalism you show our patients.

Not to be forgotten are the patients themselves. Thank you for putting your trust in me. I know for many, it wasn't easy. You would show up at my office, worried that I would dismiss you like other physicians had. It takes a lot of courage to enter the breach one more time. Some of you were angry, thinking this was going to be another waste of time. Thank you for giving me a chance.

Last but not least I would like to thank MicroGen Dx and Paratek Pharmaceuticals for not only their financial support in bringing about this book, but also your dedication to helping patients with your products. Thank you.

About the Author

Dr. Andrew Pugliese, MD, is a triple-boarded physician in Infectious Disease, Internal Medicine, and Sleep who has spent nearly the last thirty years understanding and helping people with chronic sinusitis. Relocating from NYC in the mid-nineties to metro Atlanta was an eye-opening experience seeing the number of people who suffered from chronic sinusitis. Early on, he recognized that chronic sinusitis was a multi-factorial illness, and identifying the underlying risk factors was key in helping patients with chronic sinusitis.

Page Blank Intentionally

Table of Contents

Foreword

It is with great pride and admiration that I introduce this invaluable work on the management of chronic sinusitis. Studied and written by a colleague and dear friend. I have had the privilege of working closely with Dr. Andrew Pugliese for the past 30 years.

Throughout our long and fruitful partnership, I have consistently been impressed by his unwavering commitment to his craft, his deep understanding of the complexities of chronic sinusitis, and his relentless pursuit of excellence. His expertise in this field is unmatched, and his passion for improving patient outcomes is evident on every page of this book.

Chronic sinusitis is a condition that affects millions, often leading to significant discomfort and a diminished quality of life. Yet, with his comprehensive approach, combining the latest research with practical, real-world applications, this book offers a beacon of hope to both practitioners and patients alike. It serves not only as a guide but as a testament to his dedication to advancing the field of sinusitis management. He has progressed the management of chronic sinusitis from the non-surgical approach to the perioperative use of antibiotics for more effective patient outcomes. He pioneered the multi-disciplinary approach to the treatment of chronic sinusitis. His success is legendary.

I have no doubt that readers will find this book to be an essential resource, reflecting the same level of thoroughness and care that I have witnessed firsthand over the decades. It is a true honor to present this work to you.

Sincerely,

William L. Powers

CEO and Co-Founder (retired)

Infectious Disease Consultants, Inc.

Introduction

A significant portion of the American population is afflicted by chronic sinusitis, a severe and prevalent condition. Chronic sinusitis is believed to affect approximately 146 individuals per 1,000, making it one of the most dominant chronic disorders in the United States, according to Bhattacharyya, N. (2011). Despite the progress made in treatment, the recurrence rate following minimally invasive surgery can be alarmingly high, with a potential of 60% or higher.[1]

Chronic sinusitis has substantial economic and societal repercussions. The syndrome not only induces substantial absenteeism and presenteeism—when individuals are present at work but are not wholly productive—but it also substantially reduces leisure time, thereby significantly reducing the quality of life. Direct expenditures associated with chronic sinusitis in the United States are estimated to be between $10 - $13 billion annually,

---

[1] Bhattacharyya, N. (2011). Ambulatory sinus and nasal surgery in the United States: Demographics and perioperative outcomes. The Laryngoscope, 121(3), 635-638. https://doi.org/10.1002/lary.21386

posing a substantial financial burden. These results emphasize the urgent necessity for improved management strategies and innovative remedies to alleviate the chronic disease's wide-ranging effects.

For decades, effective care for chronic sinusitis has eluded researchers, causing enormous issues not only for patients but also for their families and employers. This ongoing issue is deeply upsetting since it stops patients from engaging in common activities that many of us take for granted, such as attending their children's sporting events or excelling in their professional responsibilities.

Chronic sinusitis frequently leaves patients with significantly depleted energy levels, limiting their ability to engage in activities beyond the bare minimum required to support their livelihoods. After a long day of work, many patients are too fatigued to do much but drop into bed or sit idly in front of the television, unable to gather the energy for more active pursuits. This chronic fatigue generates a pervasive impression of missing out on life's important moments because they are too exhausted and ill to participate in what others consider typical everyday activities.

The continuing struggle with these constraints adds significantly to increased depression and anxiety among chronic sinusitis patients. The ongoing physical and mental strain worsens their feelings of loneliness and lowers their overall quality of life, highlighting the critical need for more effective treatment techniques to manage this draining condition.[2]

The most frequently asked question is why chronic sinusitis remains an important cause of concern despite advances in medical technology. After all, isn't it just a sinus infection? Why did the first three rounds of antibiotics fail to treat it? What do you mean, you've got another sinus infection? You had one only last month. It appears unlikely for someone to have so many infections. Perhaps it is all psychological. Perhaps counseling and antidepressants are all you need.

I can't count how many times patients have asked me if they had a psychiatric problem. They wonder if it's really all in their heads. My response is, "Yes, it is." The problem is entirely internal. You have an infectious and inflammatory process going on in your skull's sinus cavities that must be treated as a chronic disease rather than with intermittent therapies like surgeries, recurring antibiotics, and steroids.

---

[2] Rosenfeld, R. M., Piccirillo, J. F., Chandrasekhar, S. S., Brook, I., Ashok Kumar, K., Kramper, M., Orlandi, R. R., Palmer, J. N., Patel, Z. M., Peters, A., Walsh, S. A., & Corrigan, M. D. (2015). Clinical practice guideline (update): Adult sinusitis. Otolaryngology–Head and Neck Surgery, 152(2_suppl), S1-S39. https://doi.org/10.1177/0194599815572097

Chronic sinusitis is a highly complex disease, as explained to me many years ago by my esteemed colleague, Dr. Mark Beatty, an ENT specialist. The complexity arises from the fact that chronic sinusitis involves both anatomical and physiological factors. Anatomically, optimal communication between the sinus cavities is necessary to ensure proper drainage and to balance changes in atmospheric pressure. Many individuals suffering from sinusitis often describe themselves as human barometers, sensing impending rain well before it occurs. While surgery can address the anatomical component of the disease, the true challenge lies in managing the physiological aspects.

The physiological elements of chronic sinusitis revolve mostly around maintaining an intact mucosal membrane within the sinus cavities. An undamaged mucosal barrier is the most effective defense against sinus infections. A rupture in the integrity of this membrane might lead to the development of a sinus infection.

This book is mostly about the different risk factors that can damage the mucosal membrane layer inside the sinus cavities.

The takeaway is to help people with chronic sinusitis better understand their problems. It lists risk factors and gives ways to deal with them so that you can keep your mucous integrity healthy. It's also a great resource for doctors who have been treating people with this problem for years or even decades and who may feel like they can't get any better.

Chapter 1
Developing Chronic Sinusitis

Sinusitis, often known as sinus infection, is a disorder in which the tissue lining of the sinuses becomes inflamed. This inflammation can result in symptoms including a stuffy or runny nose, facial pain, and pressure. Sinusitis is a widespread condition that affects millions of people each year. Infections, allergies, and even pollution can all set it off.

When discussing sinusitis, it is critical to understand the two primary types: acute and chronic. Acute sinusitis is usually a short-term illness that develops after a cold or viral infection. Symptoms of acute sinusitis often last shorter than four weeks and include nasal congestion, facial pain, and a thick yellow or green nasal discharge. The majority of instances of acute sinusitis resolve on their own or with basic treatments such as rest, fluids, and over-the-counter drugs.

Chronic sinusitis, on the other hand, is a long-term illness in which symptoms last more than 12 weeks despite treatment. Chronic sinusitis can have a substantial influence on a person's quality of life by creating persistent nasal congestion, facial pain, and a decreased sense of smell. It is frequently related to underlying health problems such as allergies, nasal polyps, or respiratory tract infections. Chronic sinusitis treatment can be more complex, needing a mix of drugs, lifestyle changes, and, in some cases, surgery to enhance sinus outflow.

To sum it up, sinusitis is a common condition that can be short-term or long-term and treated differently. Understanding the differences aids in the successful management of symptoms while also enhancing general health and well-being.

To thoroughly understand chronic sinusitis, we must first examine the cause of acute sinusitis. Sinus cavities are not sterile; microorganisms live there naturally. The nasal passages allow microorganisms to travel from the atmosphere and other bodily cavities into the sinus cavities and then out. Regardless, not everyone gets sinus infections. Why is this the case?

The mucous membrane within the sinus cavities plays an important role. Various irritants can damage the mucous membrane, resulting in sinus infections. In acute sinusitis, viral infections are the leading cause of mucosal damage. During a respiratory viral disease, the virus causes inflammatory changes in the mucous membranes, resulting in sinus congestion, pressure, and rhinorrhea (runny nose).

Our immune systems often protect mucous membranes from

harm. However, an inflammatory reaction can be severe enough to compromise their integrity. When this happens, bacteria that ordinarily populates the sinus cavities might enter the submucosal area, multiplying and creating a secondary bacterial infection.

The timeline for acute bacterial sinus infections typically spans two weeks from the initial onset of the viral infection. Most patients experience a resolution of symptoms after approximately four to five days, followed by the development of fevers accompanied by purulent (pus-filled) or bloody nasal discharge. Fevers generally recur after several days, along with tenderness in one or more sinus cavities. In such cases, treatment usually involves a ten-day to two-week course of oral antibiotics, with or without systemic steroids. For patients without underlying risk factors, one course of treatment is generally sufficient.

It is important to note that another common cause of acute sinusitis is exposure to smoke, such as from a fire or chemical exposure. Cigarette smoke is another significant cause of sinusitis, often leading to chronic sinusitis with continued smoking, in contrast to the previously described situations.

In chronic sinusitis, damage to the mucosal membrane becomes recurrent. Chronic sinusitis patients' symptoms change with time. Periods of recovery are frequently followed by worsening symptoms, requiring longer treatment times than those required for acute sinusitis.

Individuals with chronic sinusitis also experience a variety of constitutional symptoms, which significantly influence their quality of life. Below is a list of symptoms associated with chronic sinusitis.

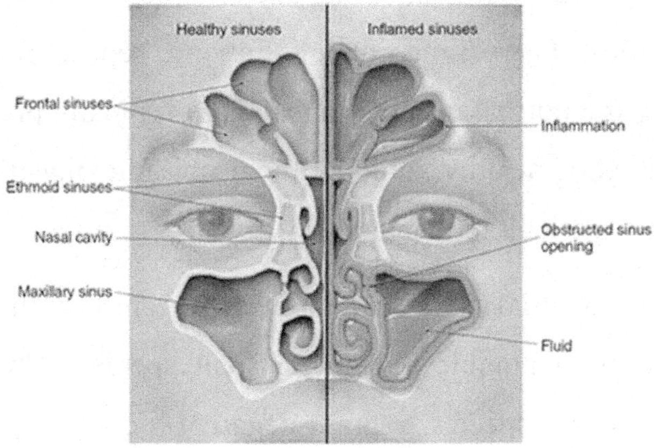

Symptoms of Chronic Sinusitis:

- Bad breath
- Fatigue
- Headache
- Sinus Pressure
- Loss of the sense of smell or Phantosmia
- Postnasal Drip and Sore Throat.
- Cough, mostly chronic
- Nasal Discharge, which is usually colored green,

yellow, brown, black and bloody

Patients suffering from chronic sinusitis frequently report experiencing halitosis, commonly known as bad breath. For many individuals, the root cause of this halitosis can be attributed to underlying Gastro-Esophageal Reflux Disease (GERD) in conjunction with alterations in the bacterial composition within the sinus cavities. Over time, and following repeated courses of antibiotics, the normal oropharyngeal flora typically present in the sinus cavities of healthy adults without chronic sinusitis becomes increasingly difficult to manage.

The bacterial flora in patients with chronic rhinosinusitis (CRS) reveals a notable rise in resistant species. These include Staphylococcus species, gram-negative enteric organisms, anaerobes, and, in certain cases, fungal species. This shift in microbial composition not only complicates treatment but also aggravates the persistence of symptoms, contributing to the chronic nature of the condition. Effective management of CRS requires a comprehensive understanding of these microbial dynamics and a tailored approach to antibiotic therapy to address the increased resistance encountered in these patients.

Fatigue is a well-known symptom among chronic sinusitis patients. In a previous study, patients with a documented history of chronic sinusitis were asked about their energy levels. The results showed that 95% of these individuals reported fatigue, with many describing it as debilitating at times.[3]

Patients with sinusitis frequently have headaches. Migraines, in particular, have been linked to chronic rhinosinusitis (CRS) owing to the inflammatory processes that occur during exacerbations of the disease. Patients with CRS also report having pressure-like headaches. This sensation is often generated by a buildup of pressure in one or more sinus cavities, which is frequently the result of blockages or compromises within the sinus systems.

Many CRS sufferers report themselves as being extremely sensitive to atmospheric changes, even claiming to be able to forecast imminent rainfall based on their symptoms. This sensitivity is related to the basic purpose of sinus cavities, which is to equalize the pressure applied to our skulls as a result of constant atmospheric pressure variations.

Without sinus cavities, our skulls would be solid, causing regular headaches as a result of pressure changes. Essentially, our sinuses function as air cushions, allowing pressure within the sinus cavities to equalize with changes in atmospheric pressure, whether

---

[3] Rudmik, L., Smith, T. L., Schlosser, R. J., Mace, J. C., Soler, Z. M., & Higgins, T. S. (2014). Productivity costs in patients with refractory chronic rhinosinusitis. Laryngoscope, 124(9), 2001-2007. https://doi.org/10.1002/lary.24687

in high or low-pressure systems. By lowering inflammation in the sinus cavities, communication between them improves, relieving pressure headaches.[4]

Chronic sinusitis is managed by controlling inflammation within the sinus cavities to alleviate symptoms like fatigue and pressure headaches. This method allows them to better manage their sensitivity to variations in atmospheric pressure.

Many people with chronic sinusitis (CRS) experience a decreased sense of smell and, in some circumstances, taste. This sensory loss is mostly caused by the inflammatory processes associated with CRS, which damage to the olfactory bulbs located near the sinuses. Furthermore, a large proportion of patients complain about unpleasant scents associated with their disease.

These odorous feelings, known as phantosmia, are sometimes described using phrases like "gym socks," "porta-potty," "garbage," and "sewer-like smells." These foul odors are often caused by bacterial colonization of the sinus cavities, namely by anaerobic and gram-negative enteric organisms such as Klebsiella,

---

[4] J Kim Thiringer, D. (2024) *Barosinusitis, Practice Essentials, Pathophysiology, Epidemiology*. Available at: https://emedicine.medscape.com/article/862964-overview?form=fpf

Enterobacter, and Acinetobacter.[5]

Post-nasal drip and a sore throat are other common complaints among people with CRS. The mucus follows the path of least resistance; when sinus cavity pathways become clogged, nasal discharge cannot flow freely through the nose. As a result, mucus rushes down the back of the throat, perhaps creating a painful throat and contributing to the chronic cough that many patients have. Furthermore, gastroesophageal reflux disease (GERD) can worsen symptoms like sore throat, post-nasal drip, halitosis, and chronic sinus infections.

As proven, CRS is a complex illness with various contributing causes that result in a wide range of symptoms. This complexity emerges because various systems may be engaged in the construction and maintenance of CRS. Identifying and understanding these systems is compulsory for addressing the basic causes and providing effective CRS treatment.

---

[5] Kern, R. C. (2000). Chronic sinusitis and anosmia: Pathologic changes in the olfactory mucosa. Laryngoscope, 110(7), 1071-1077.https://doi.org/10.1097/00005537-200007000-00014

Chapter 2

Pathophysiology of Chronic Sinusitis

Chronic sinusitis is a disease of the sinuses that lasts for a long time. It is a complicated condition that is affected by many things. One important part of its pathology is the microbiome, which is the group of microorganisms that live in our noses. In a healthy setting, these microbes help keep harmful bacteria at bay and keep things running smoothly. But when someone has recurrent sinusitis, the balance of this microbiome is thrown off. Because of this mismatch, harmful bacteria can take over, which causes biofilms to form. Biofilms are layers of defense that bacteria make to avoid being killed by the immune system and medicines. They make infections harder to treat and make sinusitis last longer.

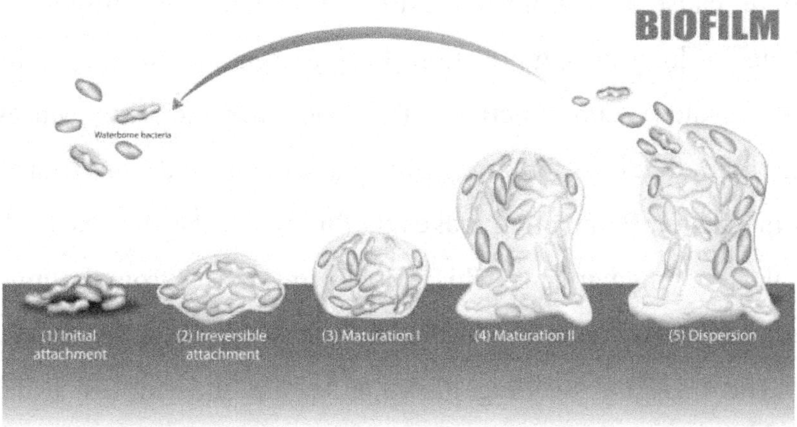

Biofilm Formation

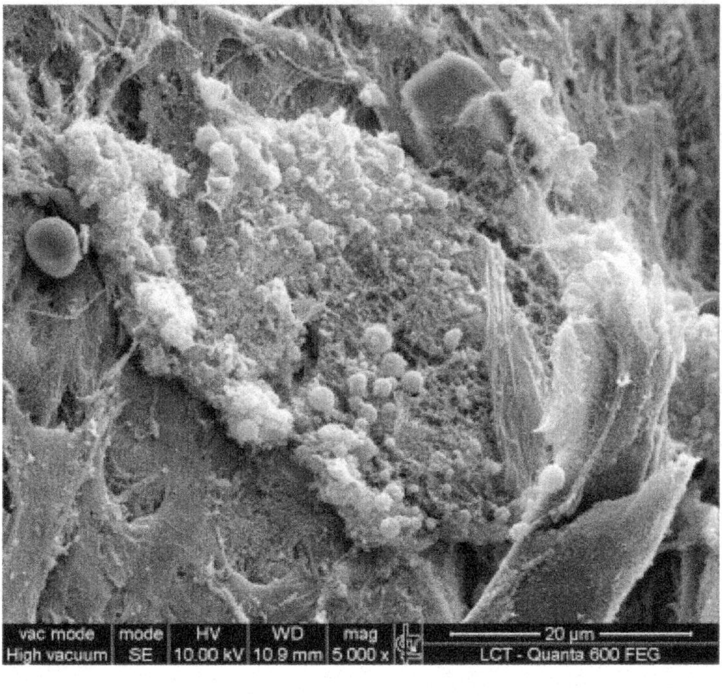

Biofilm viewed via Electron Microscrope

The body's long-term inflammatory response is another

important cause of chronic sinusitis. If irritants like allergens, pollutants, or long-lasting infections keep getting into the lungs, the immune system stays active. This ongoing activity causes inflammation that lasts for a long time and can hurt the sinus tissues over time. The inflammation makes the linings of the sinuses swell and makes too much mucus, which blocks the sinuses from draining properly and makes a good environment for bacteria and biofilms to grow. The ongoing swelling also messes up the sinuses' usual function and healing processes, which makes it hard for the body to get rid of infections and get back to being healthy.

An unhealthy microbiome causes biofilms to form and a loop of inflammation that hurts the sinus tissues. These things keep the condition going, which makes it hard to treat and get rid of.

People don't wake up one morning with CRS. They develop CRS because of one or several underlying risk factors that are not being addressed. All the risk factors contributing to CRS need to be identified and addressed properly to optimize the medical management of CRS. The four main categories involved with CRS include Anatomy, Immunology, Allergy and GERD.

Risk Factors for Chronic Sinusitis

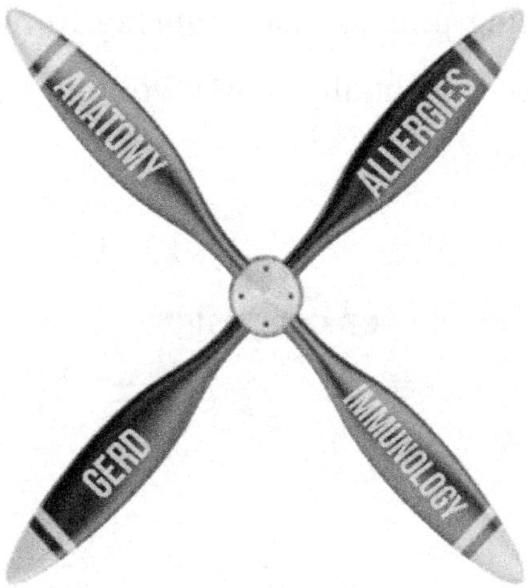

Imagine a four-bladed propellor. That propellor is able to spin properly because all four blades are intact. Unfortunately, if one of those blades is not intact, that propellor will not spin correctly. It's the same with CRS. All four categories of risk factors need to be evaluated for dysfunction, and once identified, they need to be addressed. If not, the propellor spins out of control.

Anatomy is essential. Communication between all four sinus cavities needs to be patent. If not, there is an accumulation of fluid in the compromised sinus cavity, which acts as a perfect medium for bacterial growth. (See Figure One.) The accumulation of bacteria will cause inflammation of the mucosal membrane, further contributing to compromising passages to the other sinus cavities. This will cause a wormhole effect, creating more bacterial formation, increasing pressure, and causing further damage to the mucosal membrane, potentially now involving bone, all adding to the patient's misery.

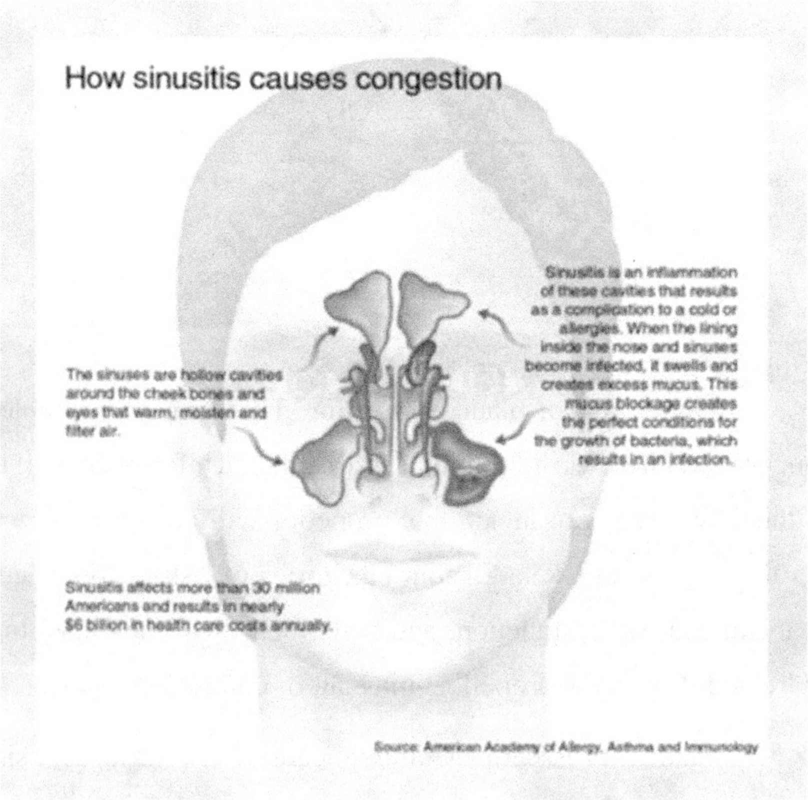

How sinusitis causes congestion

Ensuring proper anatomy is one of the major categories in managing CRS, and there are many excellent otolaryngologists out there who can accomplish it. This manual, however, will concentrate on the other three risk factors or so-called physiological aspects of CRS.

Allergies, immunologic deficiencies or dysfunction, and GERD are the three main causes of CRS. Some patients may have only one risk factor. Unfortunately, many of the more recalcitrant patients have more than one and, in many instances, will have all three.

This is where the work becomes labor intensive. It's detective work based on extensive history taking along with a physical exam. Unfortunately, many in primary care have no more than ten minutes to spend with a patient, if that much. It's easier to prescribe another course of antibiotics with or without steroids and kick the can down the road, along with the hope that the ENT can figure out what to do. This is the part that is labor intensive. Many clinicians don't have an understanding of how these risk factors can impact a patient. Eventually, many patients get frustrated and believe that what they have is as good as it gets.

This book hopes to educate patients on why they cannot get better and help clinicians understand the workups necessary to optimize their care so that they don't become a statistic. The following chapters will address the other three "blades" of the propeller individually, or as I like to call it, the medical management of CRS.

Chapter 3

Immunologic Deficiencies

One of the first things you learn in the field of infectious disease is that there is no substitute for a healthy immune system. This is especially true when it comes to CRS. Antibiotics have a key role because they stop the proliferation of the bacteria in question, but it is the host's immune system that is important in irradicating the infection. The more compromised the immune system is, the more dependency there is on antibiotics. Unfortunately, with time, we are seeing more patients being identified with primary immunodeficiencies, and fortunately, those being treated are also increasing.

Many patients struggle for years with recurrent infections before the diagnosis is finally made. It takes anywhere between nine to fifteen years from the onset of infections until the diagnosis of Primary Immunodeficiency is made. Recent literature believes that approximately ten percent of patients with CRS have some immunoglobulin deficiency. It is my belief that the number is higher, as high as twenty-five percent. I'm basing this because of my concern that not all patients with CRS are being worked up properly for immunoglobulin deficiencies. In fact, a recent meta-analysis found that 13% of patients with recurrent chronic rhinosinusitis (CRS) and 23% of patients with difficult-to-treat CRS have pooled IgG deficiencies.[6]

Like almost everything else when dealing with CRS, the workup for PI is, at times, labor intensive, and the results may not be as clear-cut as we learn in medical school.

There is a significant amount of controversy associated with identifying and treating underlying immunoglobulin deficiencies. There are many, but the most that I have seen associated with CRS are listed below.

Common Variable Immunoglobulin Deficiency

- Hyper-IgE Syndrome
- Hyper-IgM Syndrome
- IgG Subclass Deficiency
- IgA Deficiency
- Antibody Specific Deficiency

---

[6] Azar, A. (2021) *IGG deficiencies*, *Johns Hopkins Medicine*. Available at: https://www.hopkinsmedicine.org/health/conditions-and-diseases/igg-deficiencies

If patients present with a long-standing history of CRS, it is prudent for them to have a workup for immunoglobulin deficiencies. Patients in the practice who have been identified with some immunoglobulin deficiencies have seen a decrease not only in the frequency of sinus infections but also in the severity of the infections. Some patients go from having a sinus infection every other month or so, requiring several rounds of antibiotics and steroids, to maybe one or two a year, requiring one round of antibiotics.

10 FOR ADULTS Warning Signs of Primary Immunodeficiency

Primary Immunodeficiency (PI) causes children and adults to have infections that come back frequently or are unusually hard to cure. 1:500 persons are affected by one of the known Primary Immunodeficiencies. If you or someone you know is affected by two or more of the following Warning Signs, speak to a physician about the possible presence of an underlying Primary Immunodeficiency.

1. Two or more new ear infections within 1 year.
2. Two or more new sinus infections within 1 year, in the absence of allergy.
3. One pneumonia per year for more than 1 year.
4. Chronic diarrhea with weight loss.
5. Recurrent viral infections (colds, herpes, warts, condyloma).
6. Recurrent need for intravenous antibiotics to clear infections.
7. Recurrent, deep abscesses of the skin or internal organs.
8. Persistent thrush or fungal infection on skin or elsewhere.
9. Infection with normally harmless tuberculosis-like bacteria.
10. A family history of PI.

Presented as a public service by:

Jeffrey Modell Foundation | Curing PI Worldwide

CDC Funding was made possible in part by a grant from the U.S. Centers for Disease Control and Prevention (CDC).

National Heart, Lung, and Blood Institute (NHLBI) · National Cancer Institute · PPTA Plasma Protein Therapeutics Association · National Institute of Allergy and Infectious Diseases (NIAID) · NICHD

ADMA Biologics · CSL Behring · GRIFOLS · Horizon Pharma · KEDRION Biopharma · octapharma · Takeda

These warning signs were developed by the Jeffrey Modell Foundation Medical Advisory Board. Consultation with Primary Immunodeficiency experts is strongly suggested. © 2021 Jeffrey Modell Foundation

For information or referrals, contact the Jeffrey Modell Foundation: **info4pi.org**

Patients need to be aware of these signs and symptoms to see if they possibly have an underlying immunodeficiency so it can be treated. By treating the underlying deficiency, it will help in reducing both the severity and frequency of CRS.

An area that needs to be addressed is the number of immunosuppressive drugs available today to help manage autoimmune diseases. Several of these agents have caused sinusitis in my patients. In addition, several patients with underlying autoimmune diseases were also found to have underlying immunoglobulin deficiencies. Patients that I follow have done extremely well when both diseases are managed simultaneously.

Being an infectious disease expert whose professional training coincided with the beginning of the AIDs epidemic, I saw firsthand the importance of the immune system. Thankfully, with the work that has been done in the area of HIV/AIDs over the last forty years, I rarely see an HIV patient with CRS, and if I do, it's usually related to one of the other risk factors associated with CRS.

Case Presentation (1)

A thirty-eight-year-old woman came to see me with a fifteen-year history of CRS. According to the patient, she started having episodes of recurrent sinusitis after being treated for Hodgkin's lymphoma with chemotherapy.

A comprehensive workup showed that she did have PI. The most likely culprit was that the chemotherapy she received for her Hodgkin's disease had knocked out the B-cell line responsible for producing IgG, which is essential in preventing recurrent bacterial infections. At least, that was the conclusion of the immunologist who had approved IVIg therapy for this patient.

Case Presentation (2)

A sixty-year-old woman presented to me for a second opinion. Her complaints were CRS associated with a chronic cough and recurrent bronchitis. Ironically, she had a workup performed for PI and met the criteria for IVIg therapy. Sadly, she was told there was no need for IVIg therapy, hence the second opinion. Since being put on IVIg therapy, she hasn't had a sinus infection or bronchitis in over a year, and her cough has improved greatly.

Unfortunately, many clinicians today get frustrated with the approval process for IVIg therapy. It's not surprising that the first submission may be denied. In 2017, CNN reported that the director for approval of IVIg therapy was denying all claims without reviewing any charts. Of course, Aetna denied the allegations but settled out of court with the federal government on the matter.

The process is time-consuming, and many clinicians would rather not bother and move on to other patients with easier diagnoses. Thankfully, there are still those out there who will go the extra mile for their patients.

I could dedicate a whole book to the problems in our healthcare industry today. Amazingly, the COVID-19 pandemic exposed much of the dysfunction within the system. Again, how to fix it would take another book.

Chapter 4
Allergies

Allergies are a major contributor to CRS. Here in the metro Atlanta area, spring is affectionately known as pollen season. Pollen counts in March and April can hit seven to eight thousand. Many patients don't even have to be allergic to some of the pollen. There's so much of it that just the amount of it inhaled can cause irritation to the mucosa, causing damage and leading to a sinus infection.

If a patient has a seasonal component to the recurrent sinus issue, such as saying, "I only get sinus infections in the spring and fall," they need to be worked up for allergic rhinitis. Successful treatment of environmental allergies is the only thing that needs to be done to manage CRS for many.

One area in particular when talking about allergies and CRS is Allergic Fungal Sinusitis (AFS). AFS was first described in the early 2000s. Initially, there were some strict criteria for making the diagnosis. In the early days, a patient needed to show eosinophilic mucin in the sinus cavities and/or fungal elements. Today, polyp formation can be enough to make the diagnosis of AFS.

The presentation of AFS can vary from mild inflammation

of the sinus mucosa to invasive disease, where the fungus actually invades the tissue under the mucous membrane. Depending on the presentation, the management of AFS will vary. It can involve anywhere from topical antifungal sprays to intravenous antifungals in more severe cases to moving. Yes moving.

Mold is a major issue in the metro Atlanta area. The area is humid and highly vegetated, allowing mold to proliferate. Another risk factor for the mold problem in Atlanta is the dome effect.

Atlanta is a massive concrete/asphalt island in the middle of nowhere. All day long, this island absorbs heat. The warmer air draws in pollutants and mold spores.

Lately, mold counts have been high or extremely high in the metro Atlanta area, almost daily from April until December. They vary from January through March. One reason is the area's increasing population over the past decade.

Georgia has a population of just under eleven million people. The population of metro Atlanta is over six million, so over half the state's population is found in the metro Atlanta area. That concentration of people is found in roughly 8,376 square miles, compared to the whole state's 57,701 square miles. So, over half the state's population lives in almost 1/7th of the state's area, and that concentration is growing, as is the concrete island called Metro Atlanta.

Many patients find benefits when they go to areas like coastal Florida. They feel better there despite it being hot and humid. That's because the sea breezes don't allow the air to stagnate, and irritants like mold can concentrate, exacerbating the problem.

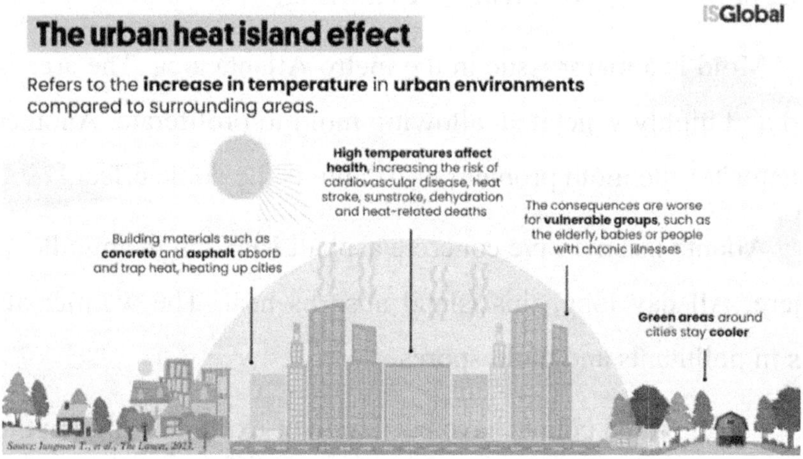

Other areas besides metro Atlanta may contribute to increasing mold concentrations that may affect patients. Valleys, in particular, may be prone to exacerbating AFS for some patients.

Management of AFS can be as simple as showering, rinsing your nose out with saline, and washing your hair after outdoor activities to surgery, antifungals, steroids, and other medications such as Singulair to help manage symptoms. The last resort, though, is relocating to other areas, usually coastal areas or out west, where the environment is usually more arid. Unfortunately, not everyone has the luxury of moving, so for them, aggressive management of

AFS is paramount.

In many instances, the most important part of the diagnosis of AFS is the history. Common statements that point me in the direction of AFS are things like I never had a problem with my sinuses until I moved to Atlanta, or I always feel better when I'm in Florida.

Some descriptive terms are associated with AFS when it comes to describing the nasal secretions they have. Terms such as Elmer's glue, wallpaper paste, sticky jelly-like snot and axle grease are just some of the descriptions I've heard over the years in reference to what comes out of patients' noses.[7]

Case Presentation (1)

A forty-three-year-old gentleman came to the office with a history of recurrent CRS. His symptoms had a seasonal component, occurring normally in the spring and fall. He was being treated by primary care and urgent care. He was found to have multiple seasonal allergies, including several mold allergies. Since being treated with allergy immunotherapy, his symptoms have improved

---

[7] *Fungal sinusitis: Why you shouldn't wait on treatment* (2024) *Cleveland Clinic*. Available at: https://my.clevelandclinic.org/health/diseases/17012-fungal-sinusitis-fungal-sinus-infection (Accessed: 29 August 2024).

significantly.

Case Presentation (2)

The patient is a fifty-year-old woman who has had trouble with her sinuses most of her adult life, and it seemed to be getting worse. DNA sequencing demonstrated that the patient did have mold in the sinus cavities. Her CT scan demonstrated that all the sinus passages were patent, and she responded well to a medicated sinus rinse with vancomycin, budesonide, and Amphotericin B. She continues to use the spray periodically and remains symptom-free.

Case Presentation (3)

A thirty-eight-year-old woman used to have minor sinus symptoms, which worsened when she moved from California to Georgia. Despite aggressive medical management, she remained highly symptomatic. The final solution for the patient was to move back to California. I was seeing the patient back in 2008-2009 during the Great Recession. Thankfully, the letter I sent to her mortgage company allowed her to get out of her current mortgage and move back to California.

Case Presentation (4)

A forty-three-year-old female patient of mine who had long-standing CRS due to AFS that was symptomatic despite aggressive treatment and maintenance therapy relocated to coastal North

Carolina three years ago. Since that time, she has been symptom-free.

Chapter 5
Gastro-Esophageal Reflux Disease

Gastro-esophageal reflux Disease, also known as GERD, contributes more to CRS than most clinicians realize. In many instances, it is missed because of the lack of complaints of heartburn. In addition, GERD may not be addressed because it's viewed more as a nuisance than a disease that can cause reversible and irreversible damage to several organs of the body.

In some instances, patients are unaware they have GERD because of the lack of esophageal symptoms. Extra-esophageal symptoms include:

- Halitosis
- Multiple dental caries in adults
- Laryngitis and hoarseness
- Sinusitis
- Asthma
- Bronchiectasis
- Chronic cough

- Pulmonary Fibrosis

Patients who present with CRS and are found to have one or more of these other findings during the review of symptoms help identify patients who may have a GERD component to their CRS problem.

Another helpful hint is the type of organisms that are found in the sinus cavities. Many times, patients with GERD-related CRS will have organisms that are usually found in the digestive tract but are now in the sinus cavities. Mostly, they are referred to as gram-negative enterics. Organisms that have been found in the sinus cavities with GERD-related CRS include Klebsiella, Enterobacter, Citrobacter, Acinetobacter, Serratia and Pseudomonas. Some newly emerging GI pathogens, such as Rauotella, have also been shown to cause CRS in GERD-related cases.

Anaerobic bacteria that normally are found in the digestive tract have also been found in the sinus cavities. Bacteria that are included in this category include Peptostreptococcus, Fusibacterium, Finegoldia, Bacteroides, Prevotella and Veillonella. There are certain species of Clostridium, such as baratii, bifermentans, and fallux, that have been found in the sinus cavities of patients with CRS. Many of the bacteria also can form a biofilm, which can make the management of CRS more recalcitrant. More will be discussed later in the book dealing with testing and treatment.

There are some concerns about why stomach acids do not kill the bacteria in the stomach. There is a lot of truth to that statement. Unfortunately, for many patients with GERD, it is not a production of too much acid in the stomach, but not enough acid. We are seeing an increase in reduced stomach acid or achlorhydria in the general population. Causes include age, stress, smoking and alcohol consumption, lack of nutrients such as zinc in the diet and stomach surgery.

Everything that has been discussed above should lead the clinician and patient to believe that there is a GERD component to the underlying CRS disease. In many instances, the GERD is worse in the evening.

Management for GERD is controversial, to say the least. Normally, I begin with lifestyle changes. Patients should try to eat the last meal of the day at least three hours before going to sleep. In some instances, four may be optimal. It is amazing how many people I see who are in bed an hour or two after eating dinner.

After dinner, snacking is another major risk factor for nighttime reflux, especially if the foods contain chocolate or caffeine. Alcohol is another contributing factor to nocturnal reflux. All of the above cause relaxation of the lower esophageal sphincter, allowing the stomach contents to come back up, which is aggravated because the patient is in either the prone or supine position.

Nicotine is another major contributor to GERD. Nicotine also causes relaxation of the lower esophageal sphincter. Unfortunately, with the recent addition of vaping, there is less damage from cigarette smoke, but more reflux is being seen with vaping. In addition, as discussed above, nicotine intake has a negative impact on stomach acid production.

Obesity is another risk factor for GERD. Obesity will increase intra-abdominal pressure, which will then override the ability of the lower esophageal sphincter to stay closed.

The treatment of GERD is controversial. The use of PPIs may help, but they can also hurt. Chronic PPI use may contribute to an over-proliferation of GI-related bacteria in the stomach that can now make their way into the sinus cavities or lungs. In addition, there are other compounds besides acids that can cause damage to the mucous membranes of the sinus cavities. These include bile and digestive enzymes. Even if the digestive enzymes are only partially inactivated by an elevated pH, there may be enough activity left to contribute to the damage of the sinus cavities, larynx and lungs.

Another controversial topic associated with GERD in general that affects many of my patients is the finding of a hiatal hernia. A hiatal hernia is when a portion of your stomach is found above the diaphragm. In many instances, the patient is told it's a small hernia, and there's nothing to worry about. To me, that's like telling a pregnant woman she's just a little bit pregnant.

It needs to be remembered that now a portion of the patient's stomach is above the diaphragm, which means stomach acid can freely flow back up the esophagus and into the sinuses and possibly the lungs. In many instances, acid reduction alone is not enough to correct the problem.

Surgical treatment for hiatal hernia has improved over the decades, but it is not one hundred percent absolute. Apparently, according to the literature, age and height are risk factors for worse outcomes associated with hiatal hernia repair.[8] One personal observation that I have seen regarding hiatal hernia repair is the length of time involved in recovery post-surgery.

There is also something called CORE syndrome that needs to be addressed because I do see quite a few patients with it. CORE syndrome stands for Chronic Cough/Asthma, Obstructive Sleep Apnea, Rhinosinusitis, and Esophageal Reflux. In many instances, the obstructive sleep apnea (OSA) component is overlooked.

The best theory of why OSA contributes to nocturnal reflux

---

[8] Ellis, R., Garwood, G., Khanna, A., Harmouch, M., Miller, C. C., & Banki, F. (2019). Patient-related risk factors associated with symptomatic recurrence requiring reoperation in laparoscopic hiatal hernia repair. *Surgery Open Science*, *1*(2), 105-110.

is that during the apneic event, the patient expands their chest, creating negative pressure in the chest cavity relative to the intra-abdominal cavity. This now acts as a siphon that sucks the gastric contents back up through the esophagus and into the throat, the lungs and the sinus cavities. There are several studies that show the relationship between OSA and GERD. There is even an IDC-10 code linking GERD with apnea. Below is some recent work in the area.

What to look for when suspecting OSA-associated GERD in a patient with CRS will be explained in detail in the workup chapter of the book.

Extra-Esophageal Presentation of Gastroesophageal Reflux Disease: 2020 Update

Marilena Durazzo, Giulia Lupi, Francesca Cicerchia, Arianna Ferro, Federica Barutta, Guglielmo Beccuti, Gabriella Gruden, and Rinaldo Pellicano provide a comprehensive overview of the extra-esophageal manifestations of gastroesophageal reflux disease (GERD) in their 2020 update.[9] This update discusses the intricate relationship between GERD and various conditions, including obstructive sleep apnea (OSA) and chronic rhinosinusitis

---

[9] Durazzo, M., Lupi, G., Cicerchia, F., Ferro, A., Barutta, F., Beccuti, G., Gruden, G., & Pellicano, R. (2020). *Extra-Esophageal Presentation of Gastroesophageal Reflux Disease: 2020 Update.*

(CRS).

GERD and Sleep Apnea

Obstructive sleep apnea (OSA) has been closely associated with GERD, with studies indicating a bidirectional relationship between the two conditions. GERD can exacerbate OSA symptoms, and OSA may increase the likelihood of GERD through mechanisms such as negative intrathoracic pressure during apneic episodes, which promotes acid reflux. Moreover, GERD has been identified as a potential factor contributing to the worsening of OSA symptoms, creating a vicious cycle that can significantly impact a patient's quality of life.[10]

OSA, CRS, and GERD: The Interconnection

Chronic rhinosinusitis (CRS) and GERD have also been shown to have a notable association with OSA. Research suggests that patients with OSA are at a higher risk of developing CRS. For instance, one study reported that individuals with OSA were 3.18 times more likely to develop CRS compared to those without OSA, irrespective of gender. Factors such as airway obstruction, reduced airflow, low oxygen levels, tissue inflammation, and compromised immune responses in OSA patients may contribute to the onset and

[10] *Medical News Today*. (2023). GERD and Sleep Apnea. Retrieved from https://www.medicalnewstoday.com/articles/gerd-and-sleep-apnea

exacerbation of sinusitis.[11]

Another study by Temprano, Geremakis, and Hinyard explores the impact of OSA, sinusitis, and GERD on severe asthma exacerbations, highlighting the interconnected nature of these conditions.[12]

The interconnectedness of OSA, CRS, and GERD underscores the importance of a multidisciplinary approach to managing these conditions. Addressing one condition may lead to improvements in the others, enhancing overall patient outcomes.

Case Presentation (1)

A seventy-year-old gentleman with a long-standing history of CRS was found to have both MRSA and Klebsiella pneumoniae in his sinus cavities per his ENT. He was effectively treated with Nuzyra (omadacycline) for four weeks while he worked on lifestyle changes regarding GERD. Periodically, the patient uses a medicated sinus rinse with tobramycin and budesonide for maintenance therapy. His last ENT appointment showed significant improvement

---

[11] National Center for Biotechnology Information. (2018). Association Between OSA and CRS. Retrieved from https://www.ncbi.nlm.nih.gov/pmc/articles/PMC5967413/

[12] Temprano, J., Geremakis, C., & Hinyard, L. (2011). Obstructive Sleep Apnea, Sinusitis, Gastroesophageal Reflux, and Severe Asthma Exacerbations. *Journal of Allergy and Clinical Immunology*. https://doi.org/10.1016/j.jaci.2011.12.326

in his sinus cavities.

Case Presentation (2)

An eighty-year-old woman who had a longstanding history of CRS associated with a horrendous chronic cough that appeared to be refractory to all treatments. Upon physical exam, the patient had significant physical findings suggesting OSA, these included a visual airway assessment of Mallampati Class IV, and a neck circumference of sixteen inches, both are considered risk factors for OSA. A home sleep study showed severe OSA with severe oxygen desaturation. Since initiating CPAP therapy, the cough has significantly improved, and the sinuses have remained clear for nearly six months.

Case Presentation (3)

A fifty-two-year-old woman had long-standing CRS where there was a significant GERD component associated with her illness. She was known for eating late at night. Once making lifestyle changes, her CRS symptoms were easier to manage. Unfortunately, the office building that she works in has water damage, contributing to mold infestation and underlying sinus issues. Thankfully, HR allows her to work from home.

Case Presentation (4)

A sixty-year-old long-time patient was initially diagnosed

with Hyper-IgE syndrome. Since receiving IVIg therapy, his symptoms have improved but were still problematic. Repeatedly, Klebsiella pneumoniae would be found in the sinus cavities, suggesting a GERD component to his refractory CRS. Since addressing GERD, his CRS has been better managed.

Chapter 6
Patient Workup

The most important part of working up a patient with CRS is the history and physical. Unfortunately, I believe taking an excellent history and physical is a dying art. The patient can give you so much information about what is going on with them. Learn to listen with your eyes and see with your ears. Many patients are reluctant to talk about what is going on with their illness. They've been to multiple doctors, they've tried multiple therapies, and here they are. Many are emotionally spent because no one believes them; they're exhausted, they're sick and tired of being sick and tired.

The first question is how long they have been suffering with CRS. If it's been since childhood or young adulthood, if the answer is yes, they need to be worked up for an immunoglobulin deficiency. Have they ever been diagnosed with pneumonia? Do they have recurrent skin infections? Another important question is whether they respond to the initial course of antibiotics or whether it takes multiple courses of antibiotics to resolve the current infection. Most patients with an IgG deficiency require multiple courses of antibiotics when they are infected.

Suppose the patient's history is more current. In that case, you need to try to consider GERD as a possibility, especially if there is a history of multiple pregnancies and the sinus issues began after the last pregnancies. Is there a history of new dental carries. Again, I think it is GERD.

If there is a seasonal history of sinus issues or an allergic component to the patient, both allergic rhinitis and AFS need to be considered. Another piece of history is if the sinus issues began after they relocated to the area they're living in now. In the metro Atlanta area, I see a number of patients who relocated here from either the Northeast or Midwest who never suffered from CRS until they moved to Atlanta.

In the review of systems, ask about sleep. Do they wake up in the middle of the night? Do they wake up coughing, do they snore, do they find themselves gasping in the middle of the night? Are their symptoms worse when they first wake up in the morning? Are they a restless sleeper? Does their bed partner complain of their snoring? If they answer yes to any of these questions, the patient needs to be worked up for OSA. Sometimes, a significant other may be very beneficial in obtaining the history because the patient may be reluctant to talk about certain issues. For example, a recent patient with CRS complained of night terrors, which are different from nightmares. In a nightmare, Freddy Kruger is chasing you; with night terrors, you wake up scared without knowing why. Sleep apnea has been shown to cause night terrors. Can you think of anything more frightening than not being able to breathe? This particular complaint of the patient shows that he has mild to moderate OSA, which has not been addressed.

Other questions to ask in the ROS are whether there are any ear or auditory issues. Both could be related to CRS and GERD. Is there DOE, dyspnea on exertion (shortness of breath with minimal movement), or asthma? Have they been told they wheeze? Are there other underlying multiple chronic conditions (MCC) associated with the patient, such as diabetes, inflammatory arthritis, an underlying malignancy, or some other chronic condition? It is important to know of these because they may influence the outcome of their care.

With the physical exam, it begins with the mouth and evaluating the oropharynx. Does it look inflamed? Is it crowded? Does the patient have enlarged tonsils that are obstructing your view of the oropharynx? One classification that helps significantly is the Malampatti scoring which assesses the visualization of the airway (see next page). If you see Malampatti Class III or IV, the patient may need to be worked up for OSA. Check neck circumference if you suspect OSA. If the neck circumference is greater than 14 inches in a woman and 17 inches in a man, a workup for OSA should be done.

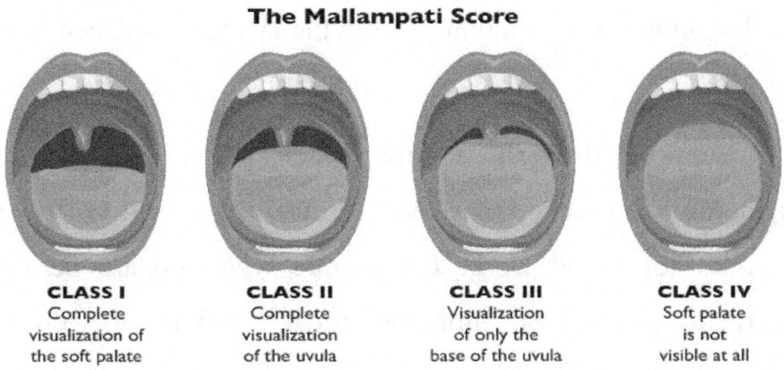

Next, look up the nose. See how much swelling there is, how much obstruction there is, and whether you see purulent discharge.

Check the ears. You may see scarring of the ear drums. Check for mastoid tenderness. There may be a mastoid component associated with the CRS.

Next, listen to the lungs. There have been times when I've heard mild wheezing that the patient is completely unaware of. If you hear crackles, the patient may have underlying bronchiectasis, which can be seen in patients with not only IgG deficiencies but cystic fibrosis (CF). Always remember that CF is a mosaic illness, and some patients do not present with the full-blown expression of CF. I have several patients who have tested positive genetically for CF that were completely unaware of the diagnosis.

Once the history and physical exam are complete, you can start figuring out what tests are needed to confirm your suspicions. If a CT scan has not been done within the last year, one needs to be done.

Suppose there is a high index of suspicion that an immunologic deficiency may exist, order IgA, IgE, IgM, IgG and subclasses for blood work. For people who you are definitely concerned about an immunological deficiency, do the pneumococcal challenge.

The pneumococcal challenge is necessary to confirm the diagnosis of an immunoglobulin deficiency. Low levels alone do not make the diagnosis. Dysfunction needs to be shown. With the pneumococcal challenge, the vaccine Pneumovax is administered after drawing blood and looking at pneumococcal antibody titers. Approximately one month after administering, the repeat titers are drawn to see if there is a two-four-fold increase in the antibody titers in at least seventy percent of the serotypes tested. Anything less than seventy percent is considered a poor response.

In addition, titers should be monitored closely for the next several months to see if there is a rapid deterioration of antibody formation. In the past, I have had patients who initially had a very robust response to the vaccine but lost a substantial amount of that immunity within a few months. In these cases, IVIg therapy was shown to be very beneficial.

Lastly, you need to know the enemy you're fighting. What are the culprits causing your patient so much misery? Routine culturing is very limited, especially if there is a delay in processing the specimen. Many organisms do not grow well on routine culture media. With routine culture media, many times, it is survival of the fittest, which may not represent what is truly going on in the sinus cavities.

PCR testing is better but also limited. PCR testing requires a different template for every organism you are looking for. Usually, most PCR panels contain ten to twenty templates, so testing is limited to the top ten or twenty organisms involved. Unfortunately, close to thirty thousand microorganisms have been identified. By relying on PCR testing, you may be missing a huge component of what is going on with the patient.

Next-generation sequencing (NGS) has been very beneficial over the years in helping me get ahead of chronic infections, which, for the most part, are polymicrobial with extensive biofilm formation. NGS allows you to see all the organisms involved with the sinus infection. It should be pointed out that the more organisms involved, the more recalcitrant eradicating the infection will be.

NGS also helps more readily identify fungal infections. Many types of fungi may not grow even if the specimen is properly processed to look for fungus. In addition, fungi may take several weeks to grow, if they grow at all.

MicroGen Dx is a company I have been using for several years to help manage many of my patients with refractory CRS. I believe that NGS testing is a necessary tool as patients, in general, are presenting with more complex infections due to MCCs. As an infectious disease specialist, the more information you have on the patient the more you can help them. There are many of my infectious disease colleagues who disagree with me, saying that it gives too much information, and it may not represent with is truly going on. My response is if the patient isn't responding to therapy, it's important to know what you are missing.

Case Presentation (1)

A forty-two-year-old long-time patient came to the office with an acute exacerbation of their CRS. The patient had been stable for several months. The exacerbation occurred in late May. NGS showed that the patient had multiple bacteria plus a fungus, Phoma macrostoma, which is used as a fungal herbicide. Phoma macrostoma has been shown to cause sinusitis and other respiratory illnesses in sensitive patients, which my patient definitely qualified for because she had been diagnosed with AFS. Recently, the patient had her lawn sprayed for weed control, and the lawncare specialist used Phoma macrostoma as an herbicide. Knowing the offending agent helped the patient avoid exposure in the future.

Case Presentation (2)

A thirty-eight-year-old patient was presented to me to help with her recurrent CRS. NGS showed the fungi Botrytis cinerea, a mold that grows on grapes. It can cause allergic reactions in sensitive patients. Botrytis can cause chronic pneumonitis, known as wine growers' pneumonitis. The patient was complaining of recurrent sinusitis. Not surprisingly, the patient lives in Napa Valley, California, and is a vintner. The wrath of grapes.

Chapter 7

Diagnostic Approaches

In order to get a good picture of what's going on with sinus problems, doctors use a number of different techniques. Imaging methods, like X-rays and CT scans, are one of the main tools. These scans give doctors clear pictures of the sinuses so they can see any blockages, swelling, or problems with the structure. For example, a CT scan can show if the sinus pathways are narrow or if there are polyps (small growths) in the sinuses. This can help find the cause of long-term sinus problems.

Endoscopic review is another very useful tool for diagnosis. An endoscope is a thin, flexible tube with a light and camera on the end that the doctor uses to look straight inside the nose and sinuses. This method lets you see the cells of the sinuses up close and can help find problems like infections, polyps, or swelling. Endoscopic review is very helpful because it lets the doctor see things in real time and can be done in the office with little pain.

Lab tests are also very important in diagnosing sinus problems. As part of these tests, samples of mucus are often examined to see if they contain bacteria or fungi. People who have nose problems may get blood tests to look for signs of allergies or other health problems that could be making them worse. Doctors may sometimes order allergy tests to find out if the sinus problems are caused by things in the surroundings.

Diagnosing sinus issues includes using imaging methods to examine the sinuses, endoscopic examinations for a more direct look, and lab tests to find infections or allergies. Together, these methods help doctors determine what's wrong with the sinuses and devise a good treatment plan.

Chapter 8
Medical Management

To treat chronic sinusitis, you need to take a mix of medicines that work on both the symptoms and the underlying reasons. Antibiotics are a main part of the treatment. These are recommended to fight bacterial infections that happen a lot with long-term sinusitis. However, biofilms can make antibiotics less effective against bacteria, so treatment may need longer rounds or certain types of antibiotics to work.

Steroids are also very important for treating recurrent sinusitis. These medicines help lower the swelling and production of mucus by reducing inflammation in the sinus tissues. Steroids can be taken by mouth, but most of the time, they are given as nasal drops to treat the sore spots directly with fewer side effects. Steroids help the sinuses drain better by lowering inflammation, which eases symptoms like stuffy nose and pressure. Unfortunately, steroids, especially given systemically, have multiple side effects and must be used judiciously, and need to be monitored closely.

When fungal diseases make sinusitis worse, antifungal drugs are used to treat them. Though fungal sinusitis doesn't happen as often as bacterial sinusitis, it can be harder to treat. To fight these infections successfully, antifungal medicines can be taken by mouth or applied through nasal sprays. It should also be pointed out that with AFS the mucosal damage can lead to secondary bacterial infections which need to be treated concomitantly.

Many different kinds of adjunctive medicines can be used along with the main treatments. For example, saline nasal irrigations help clear out mucus and other stuff that gets stuck in the nose, which relieves congestion and speeds up the mending process. You can also use decongestants and antihistamines to ease the symptoms, especially if allergens are a cause. Staying hydrated, using humidifiers, and staying away from irritants like smoke can also help your sinus health as a whole.

Antibiotics to fight infection, steroids to reduce inflammation, antifungals to fight fungal infections, and other treatments to support sinus health and ease symptoms are just a few of the ways that chronic sinusitis is treated medically. The goal of this all-around method is to treat both the causes and effects of chronic sinusitis, which will improve patients' lives.

Treatment

CRS is a multifactorial disease, and it sometimes takes multiple clinicians to address all the risk factors involved in a patient's development of sinus disease.

Once the risk factors are identified, each must be individually managed. If there is a strong suspicion of an immunoglobulin deficiency and the workup is positive for one of the deficiencies mentioned, then the patient should be started on IVIg therapy. If allergies are suspected, then allergy testing, and immunotherapy treatment are required.

When you get immunotherapy for sinus problems, which are often caused by allergies, your immune system is slowly exposed to small amounts of the thing that is making you allergic. Over time, the goal is to make you less sensitive to the allergen so that you are less likely to have symptoms when you come into contact with it in the future.

There are usually two types of this treatment: allergy shots (injections) and sublingual immunotherapy (tablets or drops put under the tongue). After a number of regular treatments, usually over a few months to a few years, your body builds up a tolerance. This can make your allergic reactions less severe and less common. It may also help ease head pressure, stuffiness, and other symptoms associated with allergies.

If GERD is suspected, begin with lifestyle changes. If the patient doesn't respond to therapy, consider a sleep study to see if OSA is a contributing factor. If a hiatal hernia is seen, and the patient isn't responding to medical management per their gastroenterologist, consider a surgical consult. Several of my patients have done well with the LINX procedure.

The LINX procedure for sinus difficulties includes surgically implanting a small, flexible ring of magnetic beads around the lower esophagus. This device helps to strengthen the lower esophageal sphincter (LES), the muscle that keeps stomach acid from leaking back into the esophagus, which can lead to nasal difficulties caused by acid reflux. The LINX procedure, which prevents acid reflux, can alleviate symptoms including heartburn, regurgitation, and perhaps linked sinus conditions like chronic cough or postnasal drip. The procedure is minimally invasive, usually performed laparoscopically, and most patients recover rapidly, returning to normal activities within a few days.

As stated earlier, treatment of sinus infections can range from topical nasal sprays and rinses to IV medications. Always try to get as much information as possible about the offending organisms in each patient and treat them with antibiotics that target the organisms. Length of therapy may be prolonged because of the chronicity of the infection and the involvement of the mucoperiosteal layer.

ENT support is essential. They can evaluate the patient with endoscopy. In addition, sometimes revision surgery is necessary. Many ENTs are board-certified in Sleep Medicine and can assist if sleep apnea is suspected.

Once the infection is cleared up, the job is not finished. As a mountain climber, you learn that getting to the top of the mountain is only 50% of the trek. You have to get back down. In CRS management, you need to continuously address the risk factors to ensure they cannot potentially cause a relapse.

A couple of pearls to leave you with are the use of leukotriene antagonists (LTRAs). The most common is montelukast, the brand being Singulair. For several of my patients with AFS, it has made a significant difference in keeping them symptom-free. If you put someone on Singulair, check a CBC after a week or so because it can cause neutropenia, a low white blood cell count, in some patients.

Always remember that no matter how hard you try, you cannot prevent your patients from being exposed to respiratory viruses. Unfortunately, without early intervention, the patient may relapse. Without oral antibiotics and steroids when symptoms first start, the patient may develop a prolonged illness with several courses of antibiotics necessary to get them back to their baseline. I call this an acute exacerbation of CRS, which is very much like an acute exacerbation of chronic bronchitis or AECB, which is usually treated with empiric antibiotic therapy to avoid hospitalizations. Maybe an acute exacerbation of CRS isn't as dramatic, but addressing the infection rapidly can avoid damage to the mucosal lining.

Nucala (mepolizumab) and Dupixent (dipilumab) are two biologics that have had some benefit as adjunct therapy for CRS. Nucala is an Interleukin or IL-5 blocker, while Dupixent is an IL-3 and IL-4 blocker. Both have been shown to help in reducing inflammation in the airway passages and reduce polyp size. Nucala is used more for severe asthma with high eosinophil counts, while Dupixent is used more for broader causes of asthma but has been used by ENTs and Allergist to help reduce sinus polyposis. I have several patients who are on either drug which has helped significantly in the management of their CRS.

Chapter 9

Surgical Interventions

When someone has recurrent sinusitis, medicines, and other treatments don't always work, and surgery is needed. People usually think about surgery when they get sinus infections a lot, have serious symptoms that don't get better with treatment, or have problems with their sinuses, like polyps or structural problems that block them.

Surgical treatments of different types can help people who have problems with their sinuses. Functional Endoscopic Sinus Surgery (FESS) is the most common type. It uses a small camera and special tools to clear out blockages and make flow better. In a different operation called balloon sinuplasty, a tiny balloon is put into the sinus openings and inflated to make the openings bigger. It is less invasive and usually takes less time to heal with this process. In more serious cases, a surgeon may need to do a bigger operation to remove damaged tissue or fix problems with the structure.

The results of sinus surgery are mostly good, and many patients feel a lot better afterward and have fewer sinus illnesses. Recovery times are different for each person, depending on the type of surgery they had and their overall health. After a few weeks, most people can go back to their normal routines, though they may need to avoid doing anything too strenuous for a while. After surgery, it's very important to do what the doctor tells you to do and go to all of your follow-up appointments to make sure you heal properly and have the best result possible.

It should be mentioned that if underlying risk factors have been identified, they need to be addressed at this time to prevent failure of surgery.

Chapter 10
Impact on Quality of Life

Not only does chronic sinusitis hurt physically, but it also has a big effect on a person's quality of life, hurting their mental and social health. Having symptoms that don't go away, like face pain, stuffy nose, and tiredness, can be very uncomfortable and frustrating. People with these physical signs often have trouble with their daily lives. They find it hard to concentrate at work, enjoy hobbies, or even sleep well. People who have chronic sinusitis may feel more stressed and anxious as a result. Having to deal with symptoms all the time can also make you feel powerless or depressed because it seems like there's no way out.

If someone has recurrent sinusitis, it can make them feel alone. Having to go to the doctor a lot, take sick days, and avoid some activities because of your symptoms can make it hard to keep up a normal social life. Friends and family may not fully understand how much pain someone is going through, which can make them feel alone and unable to get help. The condition can also lower a person's self-esteem, especially if other people can see or hear signs like stuffy noses and changes in their voice.

Patients can deal with these problems with the help of different support methods. Support groups, whether they meet in person or online, let people connect with others who understand their problems and can offer emotional support and useful help. Talk therapy can also help with the mental health parts of dealing with chronic sinusitis. Working closely with medical professionals to create an effective treatment plan can also help you better handle your symptoms, making them less of a problem in your daily life. Learning how to deal with stress in healthy ways, like through mindfulness and relaxation exercises, can also help your general health. People can feel more in charge of their situation and have a better quality of life by using these strategies.

One particular patient had three sinus surgeries. She also had underlying IgG deficiency. Faculty and friends believed she was a hypochondriac. With her last surgery several months post-operatively, she still hadn't healed. When the patient mentioned my concerns about a chronic infection, my concerns were dismissed by her ENT. Several months later, after IV antibiotics and Hyperbaric oxygen therapy, she was better; even the ENT admitted he was wrong. Regardless, the patient was left emotionally scarred and continued with counseling. Thankfully, she overcame many obstacles and is healthy now. Below is her story in her own words.

Theresa's Story

My name is Theresa, and I am a chronic sinusitis patient. I am currently in my early 30s, and for most of my childhood, I frequently got sinus infections after a cold, although I always made a recovery after a regular course of antibiotics. In my early 20s, I started experiencing chronic sinus infections that would not go away with standard antibiotic treatment. I was in the middle of pursuing a master's degree in engineering when the infections started getting worse. During my time in graduate school, as a result of my chronic sinusitis, I underwent three different sinus surgeries and developed skull base osteomyelitis that required treatment with hyperbaric oxygen therapy and almost a year of IV antibiotics. I was also diagnosed with a primary immune deficiency during graduate school. The prolonged illnesses and lengthy surgical recoveries meant that I did not have the strength or stamina to continue my studies, so I eventually had to request a leave of absence from school in order to focus on my health.

Chronic sinusitis negatively impacted the quality of my life, and I want to be able to share my story to help bring awareness to some of the difficulties of living with chronic sinus infections. Sinus pain can be really debilitating because it is right there in the middle of your head, and it is hard to get away from it. I experienced both interrupted sleep and inability to sleep due to the pain. Anytime I tried to tip my head forward or move it side-to-side, the pain increased, so I tried to limit my range of motion whenever I could. You don't realize how much you need to be able to move your head in order to go about life - I very quickly stopped driving because of the head and neck movement required to drive safely. Even reading was difficult because the sinus pain made it difficult to concentrate.

There are several subtle impacts on your quality of life, too. As with any chronic illness, a lot of people do not understand why you aren't getting better if you are going to the doctor regularly, so, sadly, some people start to assume that you are not really sick. With chronic sinusitis, especially if it is not resolving quickly with medical management, some people will suggest that you stop trying to look for medical solutions and just move on with your life. The phrases that I disliked being told the most were: "Perhaps it's just time to accept your situation" and "Don't let this stop you; just push through." While the people who said this to me hopefully meant well, their words were both unhelpful and extremely hurtful. I didn't see why I should have to accept living with chronic pain and untreated infections. And ironically, I *was* pushing myself - that is what kept me going back to the doctor, seeking answers, wanting to get better. It just didn't look like what they thought pushing should look like.

Several physicians told me that I was too driven that I was

clearly just anxious as a woman pursuing higher education in a STEM field, and that I would feel better if I just dropped out of school, as it was most likely stress headaches and not sinus pain. I lost friendships over my chronic sinusitis. Some friends just ghosted me completely, and others would only interact with me if I didn't mention my health issues. It was heavily implied by a (now former) friend that they believed I was using my health issues as an excuse to not finish grad school, because they thought I just didn't want to admit that the work was too hard or that I wasn't cut out for it. Other people would simply try to reassure me by saying that I didn't look sick, or that I couldn't be that sick since I didn't need to be in the hospital.

My advice to patients is to surround yourself with people who will let you have fun and be in pain at the same time, and don't waste time on the people who don't believe you. It still hurts whenever I think about the friendships that I lost because I was sick, but I have some amazing friends and family who stuck with me during my illness, and their continued support means so much to me. Even though I was limited in my activities due to sinus pain, we still found a way to enjoy life in spite of it all. I am lucky, because I was able to eventually find physicians who were able to help me get my chronic sinusitis under control. I am now able to manage with twice-a-day saline rinses (in addition to my weekly immunoglobulin therapy to help with the immune deficiency). I was even able to go back to school and complete my master's degree and get married!

Chapter 11

Emerging Research and Future Directions

The study of sinus health is changing very quickly. Exciting new tools and treatments are on the way that will help people with sinus problems. Biologics, which are medicines made from living things, are one of the most exciting new discoveries. Because they target and lower inflammation in the sinuses, these biologics can help people with chronic sinusitis who haven't responded well to other treatments. Also, improvements in nose rinses and sprays are making it easier for medicine to get directly to the inflamed areas, which makes them work better.

Innovations in technology are also having a big effect. For example, balloon sinuplasty is a minimally invasive treatment that uses a small balloon to clear out clogged sinus passages so that air and drainage can be better. This surgery is usually done in a doctor's office, and the recovery time is shorter than with standard sinus surgery. Another exciting area of study is making smart, implantable devices that deliver medicine directly to the tissues of the sinuses over time. These gadgets can help for a long time, so you don't have to keep getting treatments.

New information about what causes sinus problems and the best ways to treat them is constantly being found by ongoing research studies. To give you an example, researchers are looking into how genes affect sinusitis to find out why some people are more likely than others to have long-term sinus problems. Microbiome therapy, which involves putting back a healthy mix of bacteria in the sinuses to fight infection and inflammation, is also being looked into by researchers. There are currently clinical studies going on to see how well these new technologies and treatments work. This gives us hope that in the near future, sinus care will be more effective and personalized.

Finally, sinus health seems to have a bright future ahead of it thanks to new biologics, improved surgical methods, and new studies. These improvements aim to improve treatment results and the quality of life for people with long-term sinus problems.

Chapter 12
Patient Education and Self-Management

If you want to effectively manage chronic sinusitis, you need to know how your living choices, environmental factors, and self-care habits can have a big impact on easing symptoms and stopping flare-ups. First, making changes to how you live can make a big difference. Working out regularly makes the immune system stronger, and eating a lot of fruits, vegetables, and whole grains is good for your health and helps lower inflammation. It is very important to stay hydrated because it makes the mucus thinner and easier to get rid of. It's also important to stop smoking and drink less booze since both can irritate the linings of the sinuses and make symptoms worse.

Controlling your environment is another important part of treating sinusitis. Lessening your exposure to toxins and allergens can help keep your sinuses from getting swollen. To do this, you should keep your home clean and free of dust, use air purifiers to get rid of allergens, and stay away from things like pollen, cat dander, and strong smells. It's also important to keep an eye on the humidity level inside. A fan can help keep the air moist, which is good for keeping sinus linings healthy, especially in dry places or during the winter. Too much humidity isn't good either. It could proliferate mold production. If a patient's home has a humidity level greater than fifty percent, I usually suggest using a dehumidifier, if their symptoms aren't well managed. For most of my patients, I have them try to keep the humidity just under fifty percent.

Self-care strategies give patients the tools they need to manage their disease on their own. Using saline products to rinse your nose on a regular basis can help get rid of mucus and congestion. Over-the-counter decongestants and nasal sprays can help for a short time, but they should only be used carefully and not for long amounts of time to avoid getting more congested. Good sleep hygiene, like getting enough rest and sleeping with your head raised, can also help lessen symptoms at night. If you learn to spot the early signs of a sinus infection and see a doctor right away, you can avoid complications and worsening cases.

Patients with chronic sinusitis can greatly enhance their quality of life and better manage their condition by making thoughtful changes to their lifestyle, taking control of their surroundings, and implementing effective self-care habits.

Chapter 13
Comorbid Conditions

Chronic sinusitis doesn't always happen by itself; it often happens along with other health problems that make it harder to treat and hurt general health. Asthma, allergic rhinitis, and sleep apnea are three common diseases that happen together.

People who have asthma often also have chronic sinusitis. Asthma causes the lungs to become swollen and narrow. Both of them cause inflammation in the lung system, which is why they are linked. Asthma signs like wheezing, shortness of breath, and coughing can start or get worse when the sinuses are inflamed. Taking care of chronic sinuses can help you control your asthma better and lessen these bothersome symptoms.

Another common condition that goes along with chronic sinusitis is allergic rhinitis, which is also called hay fever. It's an allergic reaction to things in the air, like pollen, dust mites, or pet hair. People with allergic rhinitis sneeze, have itchy eyes and have a runny nose. These symptoms can make sinus inflammation and phlegm worse. This can make chronic sinusitis worse, making a cycle where one disease makes the other worse. Treating allergies properly can help ease the symptoms of sinusitis and make life better overall.

Sleep apnea is a dangerous sleep disorder in which breathing stops and starts frequently while you sleep. People with this disease often have chronic sinusitis since stuffy noses can make breathing problems worse at night. People who have sleep apnea may snore loudly, feel tired during the day, and have restless sleep. Treating sinusitis can help open up the nasal passages, which may help some sleep apnea signs and improve sleep.

Finally, people who have chronic sinusitis often also have asthma, allergic rhinitis, or sleep apnea, which makes things harder for them. To improve your health and well-being as a whole, you need to understand and manage these comorbid illnesses. By taking care of all the connected problems, people can get better comfort and improve their quality of life.

Anti-Tumor Necrosis Factor-alpha inhibitors have helped many patients deal with inflammatory illnesses such as rheumatoid arthritis and inflammatory bowel disease. Unfortunately, it has the potential to cause CRS in some patients. Several have presented with non-tuberculosis mycobacterium infections in the sinuses. One in particular was a patient on a biologic that developed Mycobacterium abscesses sinusitis, which required the patients to be on IV antibiotic therapy to resolve the infections. After therapy, aggressive follow-up with ENT and regular lavage therapy have helped prevent the patients from having recurrences.

Chapter 14
Pediatric Considerations

Sinusitis is a disease of the sinuses that can happen differently in kids than in adults, so it's important to be aware of this when diagnosing and treating them. When it comes to kids, sinusitis often has symptoms that look like those of other common childhood illnesses. Symptoms often include a running nose that won't go away, coughing, stuffy nose, and sometimes a low-grade fever. Kids may not always be able to clearly explain when they are uncomfortable, which can make it hard for parents and doctors to spot the problem early.

Finding sinusitis in kids is harder than finding it in adults. A lot of kids get colds and respiratory infections, which have some of the same signs as sinusitis. It takes a careful examination to tell the difference between a simple cold and sinusitis. Sinusitis can be diagnosed if the symptoms last longer than ten days, get worse after getting better at first, or are very bad, like having a high fever and thick, colored mucus coming out of your nose. Also, imaging tests like X-rays aren't as accurate on kids because their sinuses are still growing, so clinical opinion is very important.

The goal of treating pediatric sinusitis is to ease the symptoms and get rid of the illness or inflammation that is causing them. As a first step in treatment, people often use saline nose sprays to help get rid of mucus, drink a lot of water, and rest. Antibiotics may be given to people with bacterial sinusitis, but they are used carefully so that people don't get too much medicine. If allergies make sinusitis worse, taking antihistamines or nasal corticosteroids can help control the allergens that cause it. Making sure the child cleans their nose regularly and stays away from irritating things like smoke can also help stop episodes from happening again. If the problem is severe or doesn't go away, you may need to see an expert, like a pediatric ENT, for more tests and treatment.

Knowing these things about kids can ensure that sinusitis in kids is noticed and treated correctly, which speeds up recovery and avoids problems.

Chapter 15
Case Studies and Clinical Pearls

Understanding chronic sinusitis through cases from real life can help you figure out how to treat it. Let's look at some in-depth case studies and pull out some key clinical pearls, which are useful tips for both patients and healthcare professionals.

Case Study 1: Jane's Persistent Sinus Infections

Jane, a 35-year-old woman, had sinus problems over and over again for years. Even after taking medicines more than once, her symptoms would always come back. A thorough test showed that Jane had a deviated septum, which was making it hard for her sinuses to drain. After some small surgery to fix the septum and a regular routine of nasal irrigation, Jane felt a lot better.

Clinical Pearl: Problems with the structure, like a deviated septum, are often the cause of recurrent sinusitis that no one knows about. Fixing these problems can lead to long-term progress.

Case Study 2: Mark's Allergic Reactions

Mark, a 42-year-old man, had sinusitis all the time, and it seemed to get worse in the spring and fall. It turned out that Mark was very allergic to pollen and dust mites after more research. His sinusitis symptoms got a lot better with a mix of allergy management techniques, such as antihistamines, nasal corticosteroids, and steps to avoid allergens.

Clinical Pearl: Finding and treating underlying allergies is an important part of treating chronic sinusitis, especially when symptoms change with the seasons or are caused by certain allergens.

Case Study 3: Lisa's Biofilm Battle

Lisa, a 28-year-old patient, had sinusitis that wouldn't go away with regular antibiotics. Her doctor thought biofilm was forming and suggested that she take antibiotics along with a biofilm-disrupting drug. Together, this targeted method and regular sinus irrigation helped get rid of the infection. N-acetyl-cystine is one product that I use in sinus lavage where biofilm is a concern.

Clinical Pearl: Antibiotics can't always kill germs in biofilms, making infection treatment more difficult. A multifaceted method that targets biofilms may be better.

One antibiotic in particular that has been shown to help

disrupt biofilm formation is telavancin, an intravenous antibiotic that works against gram-positive bacteria such as staphylococcus and enterococcus. In several of the more severe cases of CRS involving organisms such as MRSA, telavancin was an integral part of eradicating the patient's infection.

Important clinical insights and useful tips:

1. Nasal Irrigation: Regularly rinsing your nose with saline solution can help remove mucus and reduce swelling, which can help many people feel better.
2. Changes to your lifestyle: Staying hydrated, staying away from known allergens and irritants, and using humidifiers can all help keep your lungs healthy.
3. Comprehensive Diagnosis: A full examination, including imaging studies when needed, can find structural problems and identify risk factors to help doctors figure out better ways to treat them.
4. Holistic Approach: For people with chronic sinusitis, the best results can come from a combination of medical treatments that address all the risk factors contributing to the patient's CRS, changes to their lifestyle, and, when necessary, surgery.

These case studies and clinical pearls show how important it is to have individualized treatment plans and a complete plan for dealing with chronic sinusitis. By addressing both the symptoms and the underlying causes, patients can better understand their situation and live better lives.

Testimonials and Endorsements

Leigh Kneer

Relocating down south to Atlanta for a new job after spending my entire life up north created a number of challenges, the greatest of which was dealing with the many allergens in the new climate and the sinus issues that immediately resulted. I experienced one sinus infection after another, seeing one doctor after another. However, all seemed to take the same approach, which did not provide me with the relief I so desperately needed.

Fortunately, one day while sitting in the notorious Atlanta traffic, I spotted a billboard about a Sinus Institute that advertised a new approach to addressing sinus issues. Although skeptical at first, after staring at that billboard for a couple of weeks, I decided I had nothing to lose and went in to see Dr. Pugliese. It was one of the best decisions I ever made, as his approach finally provided me with the relief I needed. The rest was history. Hard to believe that was over 25 years ago!

Thanks,

Leigh Kneer

Zachery Brice

Back in 2003, I was on the road about 80% of the week. Every time I came back to Atlanta, my allergies drove me crazy. I had issues with breathing, headaches, and nasal congestion. I went from doctor to doctor trying to resolve this issue. Then someone recommended I see Dr. Pugliese, who was an Infectious Disease Specialist.

Dr. Pugliese and his office put me through a series of tests and determined I had a serious sinus infection. He put me on antibiotics and a series of shots, which had an immediate impact on my condition. To ensure long-term relief, Dr. Pugliese had a series of X-rays of my esophagus and stomach conducted. I had to undergo a barium swallow test, which helps things show up better on X-rays. I had severe reflux. As a result of the testing, I had to get a PICC line placed and give myself intravenous antibiotics twice a day. The amount of testing Dr. Pugliese and his office conducted gave me comfort in their conclusions and recommendations for treatment. I was then referred to an allergist for allergy immunotherapy.

Are all of my allergy conditions gone? No, but they are so minor compared to how I felt prior to Dr. Pugliese's treatments.

Zachery Brice

Dr. Lester Cole, PhD

In July 2014, I had had enough. Since my return from deployment to Southeast Asia in 1972 during the Vietnam War, I had struggled with chronic sinus infections. As part of my military discharge disability, I was a frequent visitor to the VA, numerous ENTs, Infectious Disease Specialists, and PCP physicians seeking relief from frequent infections. Nothing ever really worked. By 2014, I was having sinus infections requiring antibiotics, steroids, and nasal sprays on an ongoing basis. At that time, I had been treated six times for sinus infections in less than a year. That is when a colleague referred me to Dr. Pugliese.

I needed to do something as my overall health was deteriorating. From the minute Dr. Pugliese walked into the room, I felt my hope returning. While placing me back on steroids, antibiotics, and nasal sprays, he informed me of an experimental treatment he used, noting that the testing was not covered by insurance. I gave him the go-ahead. He took cultures of my sinus and sent them off to be analyzed. A couple of weeks later, the results were back, and the culprits causing the problem were identified.

Dr. Pugliese then worked with a compounding company to develop a targeted nasal spray for my specific molds, fungi, and infections that had taken up residence in my sinuses. I began the treatment, administering the compound twice a day for a month, and returned for an assessment. My symptoms had completely resolved. I continued the twice-daily administration for another month, returned to report the complete cessation of all symptoms, and then administered the compound once a day for the next month, going to PRN at the first sign of symptoms returning.

That was over a decade ago, and I am thrilled to report that I have not had a single sinus infection, antibiotic, or steroid (except for COVID treatment) during that period. At 73, I cannot explain the positive impact this treatment has had on my overall health and well-being. I cannot imagine where I would have been had I not found Dr. Pugliese. He is certainly a dying breed.

Dr. Lester Cole, PhD

Amy Rios

I am extremely fortunate to have been one of Dr. Pugliese's patients for 21 years. As a result of my first sinus surgery in 2003, I was diagnosed with an acute Maxillary sinus infection. After multiple oral antibiotics and a CT scan my ENT referred me to Dr. Pugliese, from whom I received infectious disease expertise and very specialized care for my individual needs.

Following my first visit and PICC line, which cured the infection, Dr. Pugliese has followed up on my health and continued to be my trusted physician of choice. After experiencing additional sinus infections, he was able to run blood tests to determine a deficiency in my gamma globulin levels. Dr. Pugliese reviewed my results and was able to prescribe and administer an intravenous immune globulin treatment, which is infused every four weeks at a titrated rate.

Effective with Dr. P's diagnosis (CVID) and the beginning of my treatment, I can successfully maintain a healthy lifestyle. Of course, as a person with a compromised immune system I continue to be cautious with my surroundings, but my quality of life has seen a huge improvement. I am now able to function as a healthy woman with increased energy and can spend very precious time with friends and family, that may have been difficult before my diagnosis/ treatment.

Since my very first visit with Infectious Disease Consultants, he and his staff have made me feel so special and like part of the IDC family. I'm forever grateful to Dr. Pugliese and his practice for so many years of specialized care and his expertise that has allowed my continued health and happiness!

Made in the USA
Monee, IL
04 November 2026

67381380R00056